I0106223

From Fat to Fit

In 90 Days

A Fitness Journal

By

Onedia Gage, Ph. D.

Scriptures

So God created mankind in His own image, in the image
Of God He created them; male and female He created them.

Genesis 1:27

No, in all things we are more than conquerors through Him who loved us.

Romans 8:37

Consider it pure joy, my brothers and sisters, whenever you face trials of many kinds,
because you know that the testing of your faith produces perseverance.

James 1:2-3

Dedication

For those of us who cannot lose weight

And maintain a fitness regimen that is

Designed for healthy and wholesome

Body and life

Jordan and Nehemiah

Your athleticism inspires me

Thank you for helping me reach my goals

More Books by Onedia N. Gage, Ph. D.

Are You Ready for 9th Grade . . . Again? A Family's Guide to Success
As We Grow Together Daily Devotional for Expectant Couples
As We Grow Together Prayer Journal for Expectant Couples
As We Grow Together: Workbook for Expectant Couples Her Workbook
As We Grow Together: Workbook for Expectant Couples His Workbook
The Best 40 Days of Your Life: A Journey of Spiritual Renewal
The Blue Print: Poetry for the Soul
From Two to One: The Notebook for the Christian Couple
Hannah's Voice: Powerful Lessons in Prayer
Her Story: The Legacy of Her Fight The Devotional
Her Story: The Legacy of Her Fight The Legacy Journal
Her Story: The Legacy of Her Fight Prayers and Journal
ILY! A Mother Daughter Relationship Workbook
In Her Own Words: Notebook for the Christian Woman
In Purple Ink: Poetry for the Spirit
The Intensive Retreat for Couples for Her
The Intensive Retreat for Couples for Him
Living a Whole Life: Sermons which Promote, Prompt and Provoke Life
Love Letters to God from a Teenage Girl
The Measure of a Woman: The Details of Her Soul
The Notebook: For Me, About Me, By Me
The Notebook for the Christian Teen
On This Journey Daily Devotional for Young People
On This Journey Prayer Journal for Young People
On This Journey Prayer Journal for Young People, Volume 2
One Day More Than We Deserve Prayer Journal for the Growing Christian
Promises, Promises: A Christian Novel
Queen in the Making
Tools for These Times: Timely Sermons for Uncertain Times
With An Anointed Voice: The Power of Prayer
Yielded and Submitted: A Woman's Journey for a Life Dedicated to God
Yielded and Submitted: A Woman's Journey for a Life Dedicated to God Intimate Study
Yielded and Submitted: A Woman's Journey for a Life Dedicated to God Prayers and Journal

Library of Congress

From Fat to Fit in 90 Days:
A Fitness Journal

Onedia N. Gage, Ph. D.

Purple Ink, Inc. Press

For Information address:
Purple Ink, Inc.
10223 Broadway St., P292
Pearland, TX 77584

www.purpleink.net ♦ www.onediagage.com

onediagage@purpleink.net ♦ onediagage@onediagage.com

ISBN: 978-1-939119-20-9

Printed in the United States

Dear God,

Help me lose weight! I need help to be motivated to exercise and have enough fortitude to push away from the table. Lord, help me to stop depending on food to escape my problems. Lord, I should not need to run to food when I could just seek You for needs and concerns.

You said that I could bring all of my burdens and cares to You and You would give me rest. I need to remember to do that before I drive for a piece of cake or a pie slice.

I have not been seeking You through my anxiety over work, relationships, finances, and other issues which arrive daily. I seek comfort in that food as an escape from my issues. This overeating only adds to my problems. Now, because of my lack of discipline and self-control, my clothes do not fit and my health is in shambles. I cannot afford another wardrobe and I do not want to buy new clothes which fit right now.

Lord, I beg Your help in this matter. I love You and I cannot live without You. I cannot live with this image of myself. I am not representing You well. Lord, help those who are in the same situation. We need You. I promise to stop ignoring You.

Help me with my willpower, discipline, and self-control.

In Jesus' name, I pray and ask it all!

Amen!

My Why

I am not a fitness expert. I am not a workout junkie. I am a woman who has had several struggles with weight throughout my life. At this particular point, I just want to fit into my clothes and be healthy. I created this journal for myself. I am this sharing with you because maybe you need help as I do.

I have done the liquid diet. I lost 55 pounds. This was after I had my second child. I have thought about weight loss. I have worked out. I have tried to eat well. Sometimes it works and sometimes, I drive to find my favorite piece of cake after a bad day. I will not have the surgeries that are available. I drank the vinegar.

I have to re-develop the discipline which is required to accomplish this goal. I have to remember that I cannot allow food to control me. I have allowed life and its troubles to overcome me at the table. I have to stop eating for no reason.

Confession is good for the soul, but terrible for the reputation. I am sharing so that you know that this was not a gimmick. I wrote and designed this book in two days. Because I made a decision, I needed a tangible representation of my decision. It is not a comparison of me to someone else. It is a comparison of me to my healthier, more fit self.

My goal is to lose 95 pounds. I need to weigh 140 pounds. I have a very aggressive plan and a very tight time frame. Pray for me. I will pray for you.

Thank you for joining me.

Table of Contents

Goal Worksheet

By ____________ days, I would like to have the following

measurements and the following weight:

	Now	Future
Weight	______________________	______________________
Measurements		
Arms	______________________	______________________
Chest	______________________	______________________
Waist	______________________	______________________
Hips	______________________	______________________
Thighs	______________________	______________________

Workout Schedule

	Time	Workout/Part of the Body
Sunday	______	______________________________
Monday	______	______________________________
Tuesday	______	______________________________
Wednesday	______	______________________________
Thursday	______	______________________________
Friday	______	______________________________
Saturday	______	______________________________

From Fat to Fit

In 90 Days

A Fitness Journal

Journal

What did I do well today? ____________________

____

____

____

____

What will I do differently tomorrow? ____________________

____

____

____

____

Who will I share my success with? ____________________

What will I do when I reach my goal? How will that make me feel? ____________________

____

____

____

Date: ________________ Day 1 of 90

I can do all things through Christ who strengthens me. Philippians 4:13

What did I do today—Workout activities?

____

____

____

What did I eat today?

____

____

____

Today's overall grade: ________________

Overall Feedback: ______________________________

____

____

Father God, I submit my body to You. I pray for strength to honor You through it. Thank You for what you have allowed me to achieve today. Amen.

Journal

What did I do well today? ______________________________

____

____

____

____

What will I do differently tomorrow? ______________________________

____

____

____

____

Who will I share my success with? ______________________________

What will I do when I reach my goal? How will that make me feel? ______________________________

____

____

____

Date: ______________ Day 2 of 90

I can do all things through Christ who strengthens me. Philippians 4:13

What did I do today—Workout activities?

____

____

____

What did I eat today?

____

____

____

Today's overall grade: ______________

Overall Feedback: ______________________________

____

____

Father God, I submit my body to You. I pray for strength to honor You through it. Thank You for what you have allowed me to achieve today. Amen.

Journal

What did I do well today? ____________________

____

____

____

____

What will I do differently tomorrow? ____________________

____

____

____

____

Who will I share my success with? ____________________

What will I do when I reach my goal? How will that make me feel? ____________________

____

____

____

Date: ________________ Day 3 of 90

I can do all things through Christ who strengthens me. Philippians 4:13

What did I do today—Workout activities?

____

____

____

What did I eat today?

____

____

____

Today's overall grade: ________________

Overall Feedback: ______________________________

____

____

Father God, I submit my body to You. I pray for strength to honor You through it. Thank You for what you have allowed me to achieve today. Amen.

Journal

What did I do well today? ____

____

____

____

____

What will I do differently tomorrow? _____________________________________

____

____

____

____

Who will I share my success with? ____

What will I do when I reach my goal? How will that make me feel? ______________

____

____

____

Date: ________________ Day 4 of 90

I can do all things through Christ who strengthens me. Philippians 4:13

What did I do today—Workout activities?

____

____

____

What did I eat today?

____

____

____

Today's overall grade: ________________

Overall Feedback: ______________________________

____

____

Father God, I submit my body to You. I pray for strength to honor You through it. Thank You for what you have allowed me to achieve today. Amen.

Journal

What did I do well today? ______________________________

____

____

____

____

What will I do differently tomorrow? ______________________________

____

____

____

____

Who will I share my success with? ______________________________

What will I do when I reach my goal? How will that make me feel? ______________________________

____

____

____

Date: ________________ Day 5 of 90

I can do all things through Christ who strengthens me. Philippians 4:13

What did I do today—Workout activities?

____

____

____

What did I eat today?

____

____

____

Today's overall grade: ________________

Overall Feedback: ______________________________

____

____

Father God, I submit my body to You. I pray for strength to honor You through it. Thank You for what you have allowed me to achieve today. Amen.

Journal

What did I do well today? ______________________________

____

____

____

____

What will I do differently tomorrow? ______________________________

____

____

____

____

Who will I share my success with? ______________________________

What will I do when I reach my goal? How will that make me feel? ______________________________

____

____

____

Date: ______________ Day 6 of 90

I can do all things through Christ who strengthens me. Philippians 4:13

What did I do today—Workout activities?

___

___

___

What did I eat today?

___

___

___

Today's overall grade: ______________

Overall Feedback: ______________

___

___

Father God, I submit my body to You. I pray for strength to honor You through it. Thank You for what you have allowed me to achieve today. Amen.

Journal

What did I do well today? ______________________________

____

____

____

____

What will I do differently tomorrow? ______________________________

____

____

____

____

Who will I share my success with? ______________________________

What will I do when I reach my goal? How will that make me feel? ______________________________

____

____

____

Date: ______________ Day 7 of 90

I can do all things through Christ who strengthens me. Philippians 4:13

What did I do today—Workout activities?

___

___

___

What did I eat today?

___

___

___

Today's overall grade: ______________

Overall Feedback: ______________

___

___

Father God, I submit my body to You. I pray for strength to honor You through it. Thank You for what you have allowed me to achieve today. Amen.

Journal

What did I do well today? ____

____

____

____

____

What will I do differently tomorrow? ______________________________

____

____

____

____

Who will I share my success with? ________________________________

What will I do when I reach my goal? How will that make me feel? __________

____

____

____

Date: ________________ Day 8 of 90

Do you not know that your bodies are temples of the Holy Spirit? 1 Corinthians 9:19

What did I do today—Workout activities?

____

____

____

What did I eat today?

____

____

____

Today's overall grade: ________________

Overall Feedback: ______________________________

____

____

Father God, I submit my body to You. I pray for strength to honor You through it. Thank You for what you have allowed me to achieve today. Amen.

Journal

What did I do well today? ________________________________

____

____

____

____

What will I do differently tomorrow? ________________________

____

____

____

____

Who will I share my success with? ________________________

What will I do when I reach my goal? How will that make me feel? ______________

____

____

____

Date: ________________ Day 9 of 90

Do you not know that your bodies are temples of the Holy Spirit? 1 Corinthians 9:19

What did I do today—Workout activities?

____

____

____

What did I eat today?

____

____

____

Today's overall grade: ________________

Overall Feedback: ______________________________

____

____

Father God, I submit my body to You. I pray for strength to honor You through it. Thank You for what you have allowed me to achieve today. Amen.

Journal

What did I do well today? ____

____

____

____

____

What will I do differently tomorrow? _______________________________________

____

____

____

____

Who will I share my success with? ____

What will I do when I reach my goal? How will that make me feel? ___________________

____

____

____

Date: ________________ Day 10 of 90

Do you not know that your bodies are temples of the Holy Spirit? 1 Corinthians 9:19

What did I do today—Workout activities?

____

____

____

What did I eat today?

____

____

____

Today's overall grade: ________________

Overall Feedback: ______________________________

____

____

Father God, I submit my body to You. I pray for strength to honor You through it. Thank You for what you have allowed me to achieve today. Amen.

Journal

What did I do well today? ____________________

____

____

____

____

What will I do differently tomorrow? ____________________

____

____

____

____

Who will I share my success with? ____________________

What will I do when I reach my goal? How will that make me feel? ____________________

____

____

____

Date: ________________ Day 11 of 90

Do you not know that your bodies are temples of the Holy Spirit? 1 Corinthians 9:19

What did I do today—Workout activities?

____

____

____

What did I eat today?

____

____

____

Today's overall grade: ________________

Overall Feedback: ______________________________

____

____

Father God, I submit my body to You. I pray for strength to honor You through it. Thank You for what you have allowed me to achieve today. Amen.

Journal

What did I do well today? ______________________________

What will I do differently tomorrow? ______________________________

Who will I share my success with? ______________________________

What will I do when I reach my goal? How will that make me feel? ______________________________

Date: ________________ Day 12 of 90

Do you not know that your bodies are temples of the Holy Spirit? 1 Corinthians 9:19

What did I do today—Workout activities?

____

____

____

What did I eat today?

____

____

____

Today's overall grade: ________________

Overall Feedback: ____

____

____

Father God, I submit my body to You. I pray for strength to honor You through it. Thank You for what you have allowed me to achieve today. Amen.

Journal

What did I do well today? ______________________________

____

____

____

____

What will I do differently tomorrow? ______________________________

____

____

____

____

Who will I share my success with? ______________________________

What will I do when I reach my goal? How will that make me feel? ______________________________

____

____

____

Date: ________________ Day 13 of 90

Do you not know that your bodies are temples of the Holy Spirit? 1 Corinthians 9:19

What did I do today—Workout activities?

____

____

____

What did I eat today?

____

____

____

Today's overall grade: ________________

Overall Feedback: ______________________________

____

____

Father God, I submit my body to You. I pray for strength to honor You through it. Thank You for what you have allowed me to achieve today. Amen.

Journal

What did I do well today? ______

What will I do differently tomorrow? ______

Who will I share my success with? ______

What will I do when I reach my goal? How will that make me feel? ______

Date: ________________ Day 14 of 90

Do you not know that your bodies are temples of the Holy Spirit? 1 Corinthians 9:19

What did I do today—Workout activities?

____

____

____

What did I eat today?

____

____

____

Today's overall grade: ________________

Overall Feedback: ______________________________

____

____

Father God, I submit my body to You. I pray for strength to honor You through it. Thank You for what you have allowed me to achieve today. Amen.

Journal

What did I do well today? ______________________________

____

____

____

____

What will I do differently tomorrow? ______________________________

____

____

____

____

Who will I share my success with? ______________________________

What will I do when I reach my goal? How will that make me feel? ______________________________

____

____

____

Date: ________________ Day 15 of 90

Now unto to Him who is able . . . Ephesian 3:20 (KJV)

What did I do today—Workout activities?

____

____

____

What did I eat today?

____

____

____

Today's overall grade: ________________

Overall Feedback: ______________________________

____

____

Father God, I submit my body to You. I pray for strength to honor You through it. Thank You for what you have allowed me to achieve today. Amen.

Journal

What did I do well today? ______________________________________

____

____

____

____

What will I do differently tomorrow? ____________________________

____

____

____

____

Who will I share my success with? ______________________________

What will I do when I reach my goal? How will that make me feel? ____________

____

____

____

Date: ________________ Day 16 of 90

Now unto to Him who is able . . . Ephesian 3:20 (KJV)

What did I do today—Workout activities?

____

____

____

What did I eat today?

____

____

____

Today's overall grade: ________________

Overall Feedback: ______________________________

____

____

Father God, I submit my body to You. I pray for strength to honor You through it. Thank You for what you have allowed me to achieve today. Amen.

Journal

What did I do well today? ______________________________

____

____

____

____

What will I do differently tomorrow? ______________________________

____

____

____

____

Who will I share my success with? ______________________________

What will I do when I reach my goal? How will that make me feel? ______________________________

____

____

____

Date: ________________ Day 17 of 90

Now unto to Him who is able . . . Ephesian 3:20 (KJV)

What did I do today—Workout activities?

____

____

____

What did I eat today?

____

____

____

Today's overall grade: ________________

Overall Feedback: ________________________________

____

____

Father God, I submit my body to You. I pray for strength to honor You through it. Thank You for what you have allowed me to achieve today. Amen.

Journal

What did I do well today? ______________________________

____

____

____

____

What will I do differently tomorrow? ______________________________

____

____

____

____

Who will I share my success with? ______________________________

What will I do when I reach my goal? How will that make me feel? ______________________________

____

____

____

Date: ____________________ Day 18 of 90

Now unto to Him who is able . . . Ephesian 3:20 (KJV)

What did I do today—Workout activities?

___

___

___

What did I eat today?

___

___

___

Today's overall grade: ____________________

Overall Feedback: ____________________

___

___

Father God, I submit my body to You. I pray for strength to honor You through it. Thank You for what you have allowed me to achieve today. Amen.

Journal

What did I do well today? ______________________________

____

____

____

____

What will I do differently tomorrow? ______________________________

____

____

____

____

Who will I share my success with? ______________________________

What will I do when I reach my goal? How will that make me feel? ______________________________

____

____

____

Date: ________________ Day 19 of 90

Now unto to Him who is able . . . Ephesian 3:20 (KJV)

What did I do today—Workout activities?

___

___

___

What did I eat today?

___

___

___

Today's overall grade: ________________

Overall Feedback: ________________

___

___

Father God, I submit my body to You. I pray for strength to honor You through it. Thank You for what you have allowed me to achieve today. Amen.

Journal

What did I do well today? ____

____

____

____

____

What will I do differently tomorrow? ____________________________________

____

____

____

____

Who will I share my success with? ______________________________________

What will I do when I reach my goal? How will that make me feel? ______________

____

____

____

Date: ________________ Day 20 of 90

Now unto to Him who is able . . . Ephesian 3:20 (KJV)

What did I do today—Workout activities?

___

___

___

What did I eat today?

___

___

___

Today's overall grade: ________________

Overall Feedback: ___

___

___

Father God, I submit my body to You. I pray for strength to honor You through it. Thank You for what you have allowed me to achieve today. Amen.

Journal

What did I do well today? ______________________________

____

____

____

____

What will I do differently tomorrow? ______________________________

____

____

____

____

Who will I share my success with? ______________________________

What will I do when I reach my goal? How will that make me feel? ______________________________

____

____

____

Date: ________________ Day 21 of 90

Now unto to Him who is able . . . Ephesian 3:20 (KJV)

What did I do today—Workout activities?

____

____

____

What did I eat today?

____

____

____

Today's overall grade: ________________

Overall Feedback: ______________________________

____

____

Father God, I submit my body to You. I pray for strength to honor You through it. Thank You for what you have allowed me to achieve today. Amen.

Journal

What did I do well today? ______________________________

____

____

____

____

What will I do differently tomorrow? ______________________________

____

____

____

____

Who will I share my success with? ______________________________

What will I do when I reach my goal? How will that make me feel? ______________________________

____

____

____

Date: ________________ Day 22 of 90

No, in all things we are more than conquerors through Him who loved us. Romans 8:37

What did I do today—Workout activities?

____

____

____

What did I eat today?

____

____

____

Today's overall grade: ________________

Overall Feedback: ________________________________

____

____

Father God, I submit my body to You. I pray for strength to honor You through it. Thank You for what you have allowed me to achieve today. Amen.

Journal

What did I do well today? ______________________________

What will I do differently tomorrow? ______________________________

Who will I share my success with? ______________________________

What will I do when I reach my goal? How will that make me feel? ______________________________

Date: ________________ Day 23 of 90

No, in all things we are more than conquerors through Him who loved us. Romans 8:37

What did I do today—Workout activities?

___

___

___

What did I eat today?

___

___

___

Today's overall grade: ________________

Overall Feedback: ________________

___

___

Father God, I submit my body to You. I pray for strength to honor You through it. Thank You for what you have allowed me to achieve today. Amen.

Journal

What did I do well today? ______________________________

____

____

____

____

What will I do differently tomorrow? ______________________________

____

____

____

____

Who will I share my success with? ______________________________

What will I do when I reach my goal? How will that make me feel? ______________________________

____

____

____

Date: ________________ Day 24 of 90

No, in all things we are more than conquerors through Him who loved us. Romans 8:37

What did I do today—Workout activities?

___

___

___

What did I eat today?

___

___

___

Today's overall grade: ________________

Overall Feedback: ___

___

___

Father God, I submit my body to You. I pray for strength to honor You through it. Thank You for what you have allowed me to achieve today. Amen.

Journal

What did I do well today? ______________________________

____

____

____

____

What will I do differently tomorrow? ______________________________

____

____

____

____

Who will I share my success with? ______________________________

What will I do when I reach my goal? How will that make me feel? ______________________________

____

____

____

Date: ________________ Day 25 of 90

No, in all things we are more than conquerors through Him who loved us. Romans 8:37

What did I do today—Workout activities?

____

____

____

What did I eat today?

____

____

____

Today's overall grade: ________________

Overall Feedback: ________________________________

____

____

Father God, I submit my body to You. I pray for strength to honor You through it. Thank You for what you have allowed me to achieve today. Amen.

Journal

What did I do well today? ______________________________

____

____

____

____

What will I do differently tomorrow? ______________________________

____

____

____

____

Who will I share my success with? ______________________________

What will I do when I reach my goal? How will that make me feel? ______________________________

____

____

____

Date: ____________

Day 26 of 90

No, in all things we are more than conquerors through Him who loved us. Romans 8:37

What did I do today—Workout activities?

____

____

____

What did I eat today?

____

____

____

Today's overall grade: ____________

Overall Feedback: _______________

____

____

Father God, I submit my body to You. I pray for strength to honor You through it. Thank You for what you have allowed me to achieve today. Amen.

Journal

What did I do well today? ______________________________

____

____

____

____

What will I do differently tomorrow? ______________________________

____

____

____

____

Who will I share my success with? ______________________________

What will I do when I reach my goal? How will that make me feel? ______________________________

____

____

____

Date: ________________ Day 27 of 90

No, in all things we are more than conquerors through Him who loved us. Romans 8:37

What did I do today—Workout activities?

____

____

____

What did I eat today?

____

____

____

Today's overall grade: ________________

Overall Feedback: ________________________________

____

____

Father God, I submit my body to You. I pray for strength to honor You through it. Thank You for what you have allowed me to achieve today. Amen.

Journal

What did I do well today? ______________________________

____

____

____

____

What will I do differently tomorrow? ______________________________

____

____

____

____

Who will I share my success with? ______________________________

What will I do when I reach my goal? How will that make me feel? ______________________________

____

____

____

Date: ________________ Day 28 of 90

No, in all things we are more than conquerors through Him who loved us. Romans 8:37

What did I do today—Workout activities?

____

____

____

What did I eat today?

____

____

____

Today's overall grade: ________________

Overall Feedback: ______________________________

____

____

Father God, I submit my body to You. I pray for strength to honor You through it. Thank You for what you have allowed me to achieve today. Amen.

Journal

What did I do well today? ______________________________

____

____

____

____

What will I do differently tomorrow? ______________________________

____

____

____

____

Who will I share my success with? ______________________________

What will I do when I reach my goal? How will that make me feel? ______________________________

____

____

____

Date: ____________________ Day 29 of 90

Whatever you do, do your work heartily, as for the Lord. Colossians 3:23

What did I do today—Workout activities?

____

____

____

What did I eat today?

____

____

____

Today's overall grade: ____________________

Overall Feedback: ____

____

____

Father God, I submit my body to You. I pray for strength to honor You through it. Thank You for what you have allowed me to achieve today. Amen.

Journal

What did I do well today? ____________________

____

____

____

____

What will I do differently tomorrow? ____________________

____

____

____

____

Who will I share my success with? ____________________

What will I do when I reach my goal? How will that make me feel? ____________________

____

____

____

Date: ________________ Day 30 of 90

Whatever you do, do your work heartily, as for the Lord. Colossians 3:23

What did I do today—Workout activities?

____

____

____

What did I eat today?

____

____

____

Today's overall grade: ________________

Overall Feedback: ______________________________

____

____

Father God, I submit my body to You. I pray for strength to honor You through it. Thank You for what you have allowed me to achieve today. Amen.

Journal

What did I do well today? ______________________________

____

____

____

____

What will I do differently tomorrow? ______________________________

____

____

____

____

Who will I share my success with? ______________________________

What will I do when I reach my goal? How will that make me feel? ______________________________

____

____

____

30 Day Progress Check

I now have the following

measurements and the following weight:

	Now	+/-
Weight	____________	____________
Measurements		
Arms	____________	____________
Chest	____________	____________
Waist	____________	____________
Hips	____________	____________
Thighs	____________	____________

Journal

What did I do well today? ______________________________

____

____

____

____

What will I do differently tomorrow? ______________________________

____

____

____

____

Who will I share my success with? ______________________________

What will I do when I reach my goal? How will that make me feel? ______________________________

____

____

____

Date: ________________ Day 31 of 90

Whatever you do, do your work heartily, as for the Lord. Colossians 3:23

What did I do today—Workout activities?

____

____

____

What did I eat today?

____

____

____

Today's overall grade: ________________

Overall Feedback: ______________________________

____

____

Father God, I submit my body to You. I pray for strength to honor You through it. Thank You for what you have allowed me to achieve today. Amen.

Journal

What did I do well today? ____

____

____

____

____

What will I do differently tomorrow? ___________________________________

____

____

____

____

Who will I share my success with? ______________________________________

What will I do when I reach my goal? How will that make me feel? _____________

____

____

____

Date: ________________ Day 32 of 90

Whatever you do, do your work heartily, as for the Lord. Colossians 3:23

What did I do today—Workout activities?

____

____

____

What did I eat today?

____

____

____

Today's overall grade: ________________

Overall Feedback: ______________________________

____

____

Father God, I submit my body to You. I pray for strength to honor You through it. Thank You for what you have allowed me to achieve today. Amen.

Journal

What did I do well today? ______________________________

____

____

____

____

What will I do differently tomorrow? ______________________________

____

____

____

____

Who will I share my success with? ______________________________

What will I do when I reach my goal? How will that make me feel? ______________________________

____

____

____

Date: ________________ Day 33 of 90

Whatever you do, do your work heartily, as for the Lord. Colossians 3:23

What did I do today—Workout activities?

____

____

____

What did I eat today?

____

____

____

Today's overall grade: ________________

Overall Feedback: ______________________________

____

____

Father God, I submit my body to You. I pray for strength to honor You through it. Thank You for what you have allowed me to achieve today. Amen.

Journal

What did I do well today? ______________________________

____

____

____

____

What will I do differently tomorrow? ______________________________

____

____

____

____

Who will I share my success with? ______________________________

What will I do when I reach my goal? How will that make me feel? ______________________________

____

____

____

Date: ________________ Day 34 of 90

Whatever you do, do your work heartily, as for the Lord. Colossians 3:23

What did I do today—Workout activities?

____

____

____

What did I eat today?

____

____

____

Today's overall grade: ________________

Overall Feedback: ________________________________

____

____

Father God, I submit my body to You. I pray for strength to honor You through it. Thank You for what you have allowed me to achieve today. Amen.

Journal

What did I do well today? ____

____

____

____

____

What will I do differently tomorrow? ____________________________________

____

____

____

____

Who will I share my success with? _______________________________________

What will I do when I reach my goal? How will that make me feel? ______________

____

____

____

Date: ________________ Day 35 of 90

Whatever you do, do your work heartily, as for the Lord. Colossians 3:23

What did I do today—Workout activities?

____

____

____

What did I eat today?

____

____

____

Today's overall grade: ________________

Overall Feedback: ________________________________

____

____

Father God, I submit my body to You. I pray for strength to honor You through it. Thank You for what you have allowed me to achieve today. Amen.

Journal

What did I do well today? ______________________________

____

____

____

____

What will I do differently tomorrow? ______________________________

____

____

____

____

Who will I share my success with? ______________________________

What will I do when I reach my goal? How will that make me feel? ______________________________

____

____

____

Date: ________________ Day 36 of 90

"Come to Me, all who are weary and heavy-laden, and I will give you rest." Matthew 11:28

What did I do today—Workout activities?

____

____

____

What did I eat today?

____

____

____

Today's overall grade: ________________

Overall Feedback: ______________________________

____

____

Father God, I submit my body to You. I pray for strength to honor You through it. Thank You for what you have allowed me to achieve today. Amen.

Journal

What did I do well today? ______________________________

____

____

____

____

What will I do differently tomorrow? ______________________________

____

____

____

____

Who will I share my success with? ______________________________

What will I do when I reach my goal? How will that make me feel? ______________________________

____

____

____

Date: ________________ Day 37 of 90

"Come to Me, all who are weary and heavy-laden, and I will give you rest." Matthew 11:28

What did I do today—Workout activities?

____

____

____

What did I eat today?

____

____

____

Today's overall grade: ________________

Overall Feedback: ______________________________

____

____

Father God, I submit my body to You. I pray for strength to honor You through it. Thank You for what you have allowed me to achieve today. Amen.

Journal

What did I do well today? ______________________________

____

____

____

____

What will I do differently tomorrow? ______________________________

____

____

____

____

Who will I share my success with? ______________________________

What will I do when I reach my goal? How will that make me feel? ______________________________

____

____

____

Date: ________________ Day 38 of 90

"Come to Me, all who are weary and heavy-laden, and I will give you rest." Matthew 11:28

What did I do today—Workout activities?

____

____

____

What did I eat today?

____

____

____

Today's overall grade: ________________

Overall Feedback: ______________________________

____

____

Father God, I submit my body to You. I pray for strength to honor You through it. Thank You for what you have allowed me to achieve today. Amen.

Journal

What did I do well today? ______________________________

____

____

____

____

What will I do differently tomorrow? ______________________________

____

____

____

____

Who will I share my success with? ______________________________

What will I do when I reach my goal? How will that make me feel? ______________________________

____

____

____

Date: ________________ Day 39 of 90

"Come to Me, all who are weary and heavy-laden, and I will give you rest." Matthew 11:28

What did I do today—Workout activities?

___

___

___

What did I eat today?

___

___

___

Today's overall grade: ________________

Overall Feedback: ________________

___

___

Father God, I submit my body to You. I pray for strength to honor You through it. Thank You for what you have allowed me to achieve today. Amen.

Journal

What did I do well today? ______________________________

____

____

____

____

What will I do differently tomorrow? ______________________________

____

____

____

____

Who will I share my success with? ______________________________

What will I do when I reach my goal? How will that make me feel? ______________________________

____

____

____

Date: ________________ Day 40 of 90

"Come to Me, all who are weary and heavy-laden, and I will give you rest." Matthew 11:28

What did I do today—Workout activities?

____

____

____

What did I eat today?

____

____

____

Today's overall grade: ________________

Overall Feedback: ______________________________

____

____

Father God, I submit my body to You. I pray for strength to honor You through it. Thank You for what you have allowed me to achieve today. Amen.

Journal

What did I do well today? ____________________

____

____

____

____

What will I do differently tomorrow? ____________________

____

____

____

____

Who will I share my success with? ____________________

What will I do when I reach my goal? How will that make me feel? ____________________

____

____

____

Date: ________________ Day 41 of 90

"Come to Me, all who are weary and heavy-laden, and I will give you rest." Matthew 11:28

What did I do today—Workout activities?

____

____

____

What did I eat today?

____

____

____

Today's overall grade: ________________

Overall Feedback: ______________________________

____

____

Father God, I submit my body to You. I pray for strength to honor You through it. Thank You for what you have allowed me to achieve today. Amen.

Journal

What did I do well today? ____

____

____

____

____

What will I do differently tomorrow? ____

____

____

____

____

Who will I share my success with? ____

What will I do when I reach my goal? How will that make me feel? ____________________

____

____

____

Date: ________________ Day 42 of 90

"Come to Me, all who are weary and heavy-laden, and I will give you rest." Matthew 11:28

What did I do today—Workout activities?

____

____

____

What did I eat today?

____

____

____

Today's overall grade: ________________

Overall Feedback: ______________________________

____

____

Father God, I submit my body to You. I pray for strength to honor You through it. Thank You for what you have allowed me to achieve today. Amen.

Journal

What did I do well today? ______________________________________

____

____

____

____

What will I do differently tomorrow? ____________________________

____

____

____

____

Who will I share my success with? ______________________________

What will I do when I reach my goal? How will that make me feel? ______________

____

____

____

Date: ________________ Day 43 of 90

Without faith, it is impossible to please God. Hebrews 11:6

What did I do today—Workout activities?

____

____

____

What did I eat today?

____

____

____

Today's overall grade: ________________

Overall Feedback: ______________________________

____

____

Father God, I submit my body to You. I pray for strength to honor You through it. Thank You for what you have allowed me to achieve today. Amen.

Journal

What did I do well today? ____

____

____

____

____

What will I do differently tomorrow? ____________________________________

____

____

____

____

Who will I share my success with? _______________________________________

What will I do when I reach my goal? How will that make me feel? ____________

____

____

____

Date: ________________ Day 44 of 90

Without faith, it is impossible to please God. Hebrews 11:6

What did I do today—Workout activities?

____

____

____

What did I eat today?

____

____

____

Today's overall grade: ________________

Overall Feedback: ______________________________

____

____

Father God, I submit my body to You. I pray for strength to honor You through it. Thank You for what you have allowed me to achieve today. Amen.

Journal

What did I do well today? ______________________________

____

____

____

____

What will I do differently tomorrow? ______________________________

____

____

____

____

Who will I share my success with? ______________________________

What will I do when I reach my goal? How will that make me feel? ______________________________

____

____

____

Date: ________________ Day 45 of 90

Without faith, it is impossible to please God. Hebrews 11:6

What did I do today—Workout activities?

____

____

____

What did I eat today?

____

____

____

Today's overall grade: ________________

Overall Feedback: ______________________________

____

____

Father God, I submit my body to You. I pray for strength to honor You through it. Thank You for what you have allowed me to achieve today. Amen.

Journal

What did I do well today? ____________________

____

____

____

____

What will I do differently tomorrow? ____________________

____

____

____

____

Who will I share my success with? ____________________

What will I do when I reach my goal? How will that make me feel? ____________________

____

____

____

Date: ________________ Day 46 of 90

Without faith, it is impossible to please God. Hebrews 11:6

What did I do today—Workout activities?

____

____

____

What did I eat today?

____

____

____

Today's overall grade: ________________

Overall Feedback: ________________________________

____

____

Father God, I submit my body to You. I pray for strength to honor You through it. Thank You for what you have allowed me to achieve today. Amen.

Journal

What did I do well today? ____________________

____

____

____

____

What will I do differently tomorrow? ____________________

____

____

____

____

Who will I share my success with? ____________________

What will I do when I reach my goal? How will that make me feel? ____________________

____

____

____

Date: ________________ Day 47 of 90

Without faith, it is impossible to please God. Hebrews 11:6

What did I do today—Workout activities?

____

____

____

What did I eat today?

____

____

____

Today's overall grade: ________________

Overall Feedback: ____

____

____

Father God, I submit my body to You. I pray for strength to honor You through it. Thank You for what you have allowed me to achieve today. Amen.

Journal

What did I do well today? ______________________________

____

____

____

____

What will I do differently tomorrow? ______________________________

____

____

____

____

Who will I share my success with? ______________________________

What will I do when I reach my goal? How will that make me feel? ______________________________

____

____

____

Date: ________________ Day 48 of 90

Without faith, it is impossible to please God. Hebrews 11:6

What did I do today—Workout activities?

____

____

____

What did I eat today?

____

____

____

Today's overall grade: ________________

Overall Feedback: ________________________________

____

____

Father God, I submit my body to You. I pray for strength to honor You through it. Thank You for what you have allowed me to achieve today. Amen.

Journal

What did I do well today? ______________________________

____

____

____

____

What will I do differently tomorrow? ______________________________

____

____

____

____

Who will I share my success with? ______________________________

What will I do when I reach my goal? How will that make me feel? ______________________________

____

____

____

Date: ________________ Day 49 of 90

Without faith, it is impossible to please God. Hebrews 11:6

What did I do today—Workout activities?

____

____

____

What did I eat today?

____

____

____

Today's overall grade: ________________

Overall Feedback: ________________________________

____

____

Father God, I submit my body to You. I pray for strength to honor You through it. Thank You for what you have allowed me to achieve today. Amen.

Journal

What did I do well today? ______________________________

____

____

____

____

What will I do differently tomorrow? ______________________________

____

____

____

____

Who will I share my success with? ______________________________

What will I do when I reach my goal? How will that make me feel? ______________________________

____

____

____

Date: ______________ Day 50 of 90

I am fearfully and wonderfully made. Psalm 139:14

What did I do today—Workout activities?

____

____

____

What did I eat today?

____

____

____

Today's overall grade: ______________

Overall Feedback: ______________________________

____

____

Father God, I submit my body to You. I pray for strength to honor You through it. Thank You for what you have allowed me to achieve today. Amen.

Journal

What did I do well today? ____________________

____

____

____

____

What will I do differently tomorrow? ____________________

____

____

____

____

Who will I share my success with? ____________________

What will I do when I reach my goal? How will that make me feel? ____________________

____

____

____

Date: ________________ Day 51 of 90

I am fearfully and wonderfully made. Psalm 139:14

What did I do today—Workout activities?

____

____

____

What did I eat today?

____

____

____

Today's overall grade: ________________

Overall Feedback: ______________________________

____

____

Father God, I submit my body to You. I pray for strength to honor You through it. Thank You for what you have allowed me to achieve today. Amen.

Journal

What did I do well today? ______________________________

____

____

____

____

What will I do differently tomorrow? ______________________________

____

____

____

____

Who will I share my success with? ______________________________

What will I do when I reach my goal? How will that make me feel? ______________________________

____

____

____

Date: ________________ Day 52 of 90

I am fearfully and wonderfully made. Psalm 139:14

What did I do today—Workout activities?

____

____

____

What did I eat today?

____

____

____

Today's overall grade: ________________

Overall Feedback: ______________________________

____

____

Father God, I submit my body to You. I pray for strength to honor You through it. Thank You for what you have allowed me to achieve today. Amen.

Journal

What did I do well today? ______________________________

____

____

____

____

What will I do differently tomorrow? ______________________________

____

____

____

____

Who will I share my success with? ______________________________

What will I do when I reach my goal? How will that make me feel? ______________________________

____

____

____

Date: ________________ Day 53 of 90

I am fearfully and wonderfully made. Psalm 139:14

What did I do today—Workout activities?

____

____

____

What did I eat today?

____

____

____

Today's overall grade: ________________

Overall Feedback: ______________________________

____

____

Father God, I submit my body to You. I pray for strength to honor You through it. Thank You for what you have allowed me to achieve today. Amen.

Journal

What did I do well today? ______________________________

____

____

____

____

What will I do differently tomorrow? ______________________________

____

____

____

____

Who will I share my success with? ______________________________

What will I do when I reach my goal? How will that make me feel? ______________________________

____

____

____

Date: ________________ Day 54 of 90

I am fearfully and wonderfully made. Psalm 139:14

What did I do today—Workout activities?

____

____

____

What did I eat today?

____

____

____

Today's overall grade: ________________

Overall Feedback: ________________________________

____

____

Father God, I submit my body to You. I pray for strength to honor You through it. Thank You for what you have allowed me to achieve today. Amen.

Journal

What did I do well today? ______________________________

____

____

____

____

What will I do differently tomorrow? ______________________________

____

____

____

____

Who will I share my success with? ______________________________

What will I do when I reach my goal? How will that make me feel? ______________________________

____

____

____

Date: ________________ Day 55 of 90

I am fearfully and wonderfully made. Psalm 139:14

What did I do today—Workout activities?

____

____

____

What did I eat today?

____

____

____

Today's overall grade: ________________

Overall Feedback: ______________________________

____

____

Father God, I submit my body to You. I pray for strength to honor You through it. Thank You for what you have allowed me to achieve today. Amen.

Journal

What did I do well today? ________________________________

____

____

____

____

What will I do differently tomorrow? ________________________

____

____

____

____

Who will I share my success with? __________________________

What will I do when I reach my goal? How will that make me feel? __________

____

____

____

Date: ________________ Day 56 of 90

I am fearfully and wonderfully made. Psalm 139:14

What did I do today—Workout activities?

___

___

___

What did I eat today?

___

___

___

Today's overall grade: ________________

Overall Feedback: ________________

___

___

Father God, I submit my body to You. I pray for strength to honor You through it. Thank You for what you have allowed me to achieve today. Amen.

Journal

What did I do well today? ______________________________

____

____

____

____

What will I do differently tomorrow? ______________________________

____

____

____

____

Who will I share my success with? ______________________________

What will I do when I reach my goal? How will that make me feel? ______________________________

____

____

____

Date: ________________ Day 57 of 90

Be anxious for nothing, but in everything by prayer . . . Philippians 4:6

What did I do today—Workout activities?

____

____

____

What did I eat today?

____

____

____

Today's overall grade: ________________

Overall Feedback: ________________________________

____

____

Father God, I submit my body to You. I pray for strength to honor You through it. Thank You for what you have allowed me to achieve today. Amen.

Journal

What did I do well today? ______________________________

____

____

____

____

What will I do differently tomorrow? ______________________________

____

____

____

____

Who will I share my success with? ______________________________

What will I do when I reach my goal? How will that make me feel? ______________________________

____

____

____

Date: ________________ Day 58 of 90

Be anxious for nothing, but in everything by prayer . . . Philippians 4:6

What did I do today—Workout activities?

____

____

____

What did I eat today?

____

____

____

Today's overall grade: ________________

Overall Feedback: ______________________________

____

____

Father God, I submit my body to You. I pray for strength to honor You through it. Thank You for what you have allowed me to achieve today. Amen.

Journal

What did I do well today? ______________________________

____

____

____

____

What will I do differently tomorrow? ______________________________

____

____

____

____

Who will I share my success with? ______________________________

What will I do when I reach my goal? How will that make me feel? ______________________________

____

____

____

Date: ____________ Day 59 of 90

Be anxious for nothing, but in everything by prayer . . . Philippians 4:6

What did I do today—Workout activities?

____

____

____

What did I eat today?

____

____

____

Today's overall grade: ____________

Overall Feedback: ______________________________

____

____

Father God, I submit my body to You. I pray for strength to honor You through it. Thank You for what you have allowed me to achieve today. Amen.

Journal

What did I do well today? ______________________________

____

____

____

____

What will I do differently tomorrow? ______________________________

____

____

____

____

Who will I share my success with? ______________________________

What will I do when I reach my goal? How will that make me feel? ______________________________

____

____

____

Date: ________________ Day 60 of 90

Be anxious for nothing, but in everything by prayer . . . Philippians 4:6

What did I do today—Workout activities?

____

____

____

What did I eat today?

____

____

____

Today's overall grade: ________________

Overall Feedback: ________________________________

____

____

Father God, I submit my body to You. I pray for strength to honor You through it. Thank You for what you have allowed me to achieve today. Amen.

Journal

What did I do well today? ______________________________

____

____

____

____

What will I do differently tomorrow? ______________________________

____

____

____

____

Who will I share my success with? ______________________________

What will I do when I reach my goal? How will that make me feel? ______________________________

____

____

____

60 Day Progress Check

I now have the following

measurements and the following weight:

	Now	+/-
Weight	______________	______________
Measurements		
Arms	______________	______________
Chest	______________	______________
Waist	______________	______________
Hips	______________	______________
Thighs	______________	______________

Journal

What did I do well today? ______________________________

____

____

____

____

What will I do differently tomorrow? ______________________________

____

____

____

____

Who will I share my success with? ______________________________

What will I do when I reach my goal? How will that make me feel? ______________________________

____

____

____

Date: ________________ Day 61 of 90

Be anxious for nothing, but in everything by prayer . . . Philippians 4:6

What did I do today—Workout activities?

____

____

____

What did I eat today?

____

____

____

Today's overall grade: ________________

Overall Feedback: _______________________________

____

____

Father God, I submit my body to You. I pray for strength to honor You through it. Thank You for what you have allowed me to achieve today. Amen.

Journal

What did I do well today? ____________________

____

____

____

____

What will I do differently tomorrow? ____________________

____

____

____

____

Who will I share my success with? ____________________

What will I do when I reach my goal? How will that make me feel? ____________________

____

____

____

Date: ______________ Day 62 of 90

Be anxious for nothing, but in everything by prayer . . . Philippians 4:6

What did I do today—Workout activities?

____

____

____

What did I eat today?

____

____

____

Today's overall grade: ______________

Overall Feedback: ______________________________

____

____

Father God, I submit my body to You. I pray for strength to honor You through it. Thank You for what you have allowed me to achieve today. Amen.

Journal

What did I do well today? ______________________________

____

____

____

____

What will I do differently tomorrow? ______________________________

____

____

____

____

Who will I share my success with? ______________________________

What will I do when I reach my goal? How will that make me feel? ______________________________

____

____

____

Date: ________________ Day 63 of 90

Be anxious for nothing, but in everything by prayer . . . Philippians 4:6

What did I do today—Workout activities?

____

____

____

What did I eat today?

____

____

____

Today's overall grade: ________________

Overall Feedback: ______________________________

____

____

Father God, I submit my body to You. I pray for strength to honor You through it. Thank You for what you have allowed me to achieve today. Amen.

Journal

What did I do well today? ______________________________

____

____

____

____

What will I do differently tomorrow? ______________________________

____

____

____

____

Who will I share my success with? ______________________________

What will I do when I reach my goal? How will that make me feel? ______________________________

____

____

____

Date: ________________ Day 64 of 90

And the peace of God, which surpasses all comprehension . . . Philippians 4:7

What did I do today—Workout activities?

____

____

____

What did I eat today?

____

____

____

Today's overall grade: ________________

Overall Feedback: ______________________________

____

____

Father God, I submit my body to You. I pray for strength to honor You through it. Thank You for what you have allowed me to achieve today. Amen.

Journal

What did I do well today? ______________________________

____

____

____

____

What will I do differently tomorrow? ______________________________

____

____

____

____

Who will I share my success with? ______________________________

What will I do when I reach my goal? How will that make me feel? ______________________________

____

____

____

Date: ________________ Day 65 of 90

And the peace of God, which surpasses all comprehension . . . Philippians 4:7

What did I do today—Workout activities?

____

____

____

What did I eat today?

____

____

____

Today's overall grade: ________________

Overall Feedback: ________________________________

____

____

Father God, I submit my body to You. I pray for strength to honor You through it. Thank You for what you have allowed me to achieve today. Amen.

Journal

What did I do well today? ______________________________

____

____

____

____

What will I do differently tomorrow? ______________________________

____

____

____

____

Who will I share my success with? ______________________________

What will I do when I reach my goal? How will that make me feel? ______________________________

____

____

____

Date: ________________ Day 66 of 90

And the peace of God, which surpasses all comprehension . . . Philippians 4:7

What did I do today—Workout activities?

____

____

____

What did I eat today?

____

____

____

Today's overall grade: ________________

Overall Feedback: ______________________________

____

____

Father God, I submit my body to You. I pray for strength to honor You through it. Thank You for what you have allowed me to achieve today. Amen.

Journal

What did I do well today? ______________________________

____

____

____

____

What will I do differently tomorrow? ______________________________

____

____

____

____

Who will I share my success with? ______________________________

What will I do when I reach my goal? How will that make me feel? ______________________________

____

____

____

Date: ________________ Day 67 of 90

And the peace of God, which surpasses all comprehension . . . Philippians 4:7

What did I do today—Workout activities?

____

____

____

What did I eat today?

____

____

____

Today's overall grade: ________________

Overall Feedback: ______________________________

____

____

Father God, I submit my body to You. I pray for strength to honor You through it. Thank You for what you have allowed me to achieve today. Amen.

Journal

What did I do well today? ______________________________

____

____

____

____

What will I do differently tomorrow? ______________________________

____

____

____

____

Who will I share my success with? ______________________________

What will I do when I reach my goal? How will that make me feel? ______________________________

____

____

____

Date: ____________________ Day 68 of 90

And the peace of God, which surpasses all comprehension . . . Philippians 4:7

What did I do today—Workout activities?

____

____

____

What did I eat today?

____

____

____

Today's overall grade: ____________________

Overall Feedback: ____

____

____

Father God, I submit my body to You. I pray for strength to honor You through it. Thank You for what you have allowed me to achieve today. Amen.

Journal

What did I do well today? ______________________________

____

____

____

____

What will I do differently tomorrow? ______________________________

____

____

____

____

Who will I share my success with? ______________________________

What will I do when I reach my goal? How will that make me feel? ______________________________

____

____

____

Date: ____________ Day 69 of 90

And the peace of God, which surpasses all comprehension . . . Philippians 4:7

What did I do today—Workout activities?

___

___

___

What did I eat today?

___

___

___

Today's overall grade: ____________

Overall Feedback: ____________

___

___

Father God, I submit my body to You. I pray for strength to honor You through it. Thank You for what you have allowed me to achieve today. Amen.

Journal

What did I do well today? ______________________________

____

____

____

____

What will I do differently tomorrow? ______________________________

____

____

____

____

Who will I share my success with? ______________________________

What will I do when I reach my goal? How will that make me feel? ______________________________

____

____

____

Date: ________________ Day 70 of 90

And the peace of God, which surpasses all comprehension . . . Philippians 4:7

What did I do today—Workout activities?

____

____

____

What did I eat today?

____

____

____

Today's overall grade: ________________

Overall Feedback: ________________________________

____

____

Father God, I submit my body to You. I pray for strength to honor You through it. Thank You for what you have allowed me to achieve today. Amen.

Journal

What did I do well today? ______________________________

____

____

____

____

What will I do differently tomorrow? ______________________________

____

____

____

____

Who will I share my success with? ______________________________

What will I do when I reach my goal? How will that make me feel? ______________________________

____

____

____

Date: ________________ Day 71 of 90

"Before I formed you in your mother's womb I knew you" Jeremiah 1:5

What did I do today—Workout activities?

____

____

____

What did I eat today?

____

____

____

Today's overall grade: ________________

Overall Feedback: ______________________________

____

____

Father God, I submit my body to You. I pray for strength to honor You through it. Thank You for what you have allowed me to achieve today. Amen.

Journal

What did I do well today? ______________________________

What will I do differently tomorrow? ______________________________

Who will I share my success with? ______________________________

What will I do when I reach my goal? How will that make me feel? ______________________________

Date: ________________ Day 72 of 90

"Before I formed you in your mother's womb I knew you" Jeremiah 1:5

What did I do today—Workout activities?

____

____

____

What did I eat today?

____

____

____

Today's overall grade: ________________

Overall Feedback: ____

____

____

Father God, I submit my body to You. I pray for strength to honor You through it. Thank You for what you have allowed me to achieve today. Amen.

Journal

What did I do well today? ______________________________

____

____

____

____

What will I do differently tomorrow? ______________________________

____

____

____

____

Who will I share my success with? ______________________________

What will I do when I reach my goal? How will that make me feel? ______________________________

____

____

____

Date: ________________ Day 73 of 90

"Before I formed you in your mother's womb I knew you" Jeremiah 1:5

What did I do today—Workout activities?

____

____

____

What did I eat today?

____

____

____

Today's overall grade: ________________

Overall Feedback: ______________________________

____

____

Father God, I submit my body to You. I pray for strength to honor You through it. Thank You for what you have allowed me to achieve today. Amen.

Journal

What did I do well today? ____________________

____

____

____

____

What will I do differently tomorrow? ____________________

____

____

____

____

Who will I share my success with? ____________________

What will I do when I reach my goal? How will that make me feel? ____________________

____

____

____

Date: ________________ Day 74 of 90

"Before I formed you in your mother's womb I knew you" Jeremiah 1:5

What did I do today—Workout activities?

____

____

____

What did I eat today?

____

____

____

Today's overall grade: ________________

Overall Feedback: ______________________________

____

____

Father God, I submit my body to You. I pray for strength to honor You through it. Thank You for what you have allowed me to achieve today. Amen.

Journal

What did I do well today? ______________________________

____

____

____

____

What will I do differently tomorrow? ______________________________

____

____

____

____

Who will I share my success with? ______________________________

What will I do when I reach my goal? How will that make me feel? ______________________________

____

____

____

Date: ________________ Day 75 of 90

"Before I formed you in your mother's womb I knew you" Jeremiah 1:5

What did I do today—Workout activities?

____

____

____

What did I eat today?

____

____

____

Today's overall grade: ________________

Overall Feedback: ______________________________

____

____

Father God, I submit my body to You. I pray for strength to honor You through it. Thank You for what you have allowed me to achieve today. Amen.

Journal

What did I do well today? ______________________________

____

____

____

____

What will I do differently tomorrow? ______________________________

____

____

____

____

Who will I share my success with? ______________________________

What will I do when I reach my goal? How will that make me feel? ______________________________

____

____

____

Date: ________________ Day 76 of 90

"Before I formed you in your mother's womb I knew you" Jeremiah 1:5

What did I do today—Workout activities?

____

____

____

What did I eat today?

____

____

____

Today's overall grade: ________________

Overall Feedback: _______________________________

____

____

Father God, I submit my body to You. I pray for strength to honor You through it. Thank You for what you have allowed me to achieve today. Amen.

Journal

What did I do well today? ______________________________

____

____

____

____

What will I do differently tomorrow? ______________________________

____

____

____

____

Who will I share my success with? ______________________________

What will I do when I reach my goal? How will that make me feel? ______________________________

____

____

____

Date: ________________ Day 77 of 90

"Before I formed you in your mother's womb I knew you" Jeremiah 1:5

What did I do today—Workout activities?

____

____

____

What did I eat today?

____

____

____

Today's overall grade: ________________

Overall Feedback: _______________________________

____

____

Father God, I submit my body to You. I pray for strength to honor You through it. Thank You for what you have allowed me to achieve today. Amen.

Journal

What did I do well today? ______________________________

____

____

____

____

What will I do differently tomorrow? ______________________________

____

____

____

____

Who will I share my success with? ______________________________

What will I do when I reach my goal? How will that make me feel? ______________________________

____

____

____

Date: ________________ Day 78 of 90

I press on toward the goal to win the prize for which God has called. Philippians 3:14

What did I do today—Workout activities?

____

____

____

What did I eat today?

____

____

____

Today's overall grade: ________________

Overall Feedback: ______________________________

____

____

Father God, I submit my body to You. I pray for strength to honor You through it. Thank You for what you have allowed me to achieve today. Amen.

Journal

What did I do well today? ______________________________

____

____

____

____

What will I do differently tomorrow? ______________________________

____

____

____

____

Who will I share my success with? ______________________________

What will I do when I reach my goal? How will that make me feel? ______________________________

____

____

____

Date: ________________ Day 79 of 90

I press on toward the goal to win the prize for which God has called. Philippians 3:14

What did I do today—Workout activities?

____

____

____

What did I eat today?

____

____

____

Today's overall grade: ________________

Overall Feedback: ______________________________

____

____

Father God, I submit my body to You. I pray for strength to honor You through it. Thank You for what you have allowed me to achieve today. Amen.

Journal

What did I do well today? ______________________________

____

____

____

____

What will I do differently tomorrow? ______________________________

____

____

____

____

Who will I share my success with? ______________________________

What will I do when I reach my goal? How will that make me feel? ______________________________

____

____

____

Date: ________________ Day 80 of 90

I press on toward the goal to win the prize for which God has called. Philippians 3:14

What did I do today—Workout activities?

____

____

____

What did I eat today?

____

____

____

Today's overall grade: ________________

Overall Feedback: ______________________________

____

____

Father God, I submit my body to You. I pray for strength to honor You through it. Thank You for what you have allowed me to achieve today. Amen.

Journal

What did I do well today? ______________________________

____

____

____

____

What will I do differently tomorrow? ______________________________

____

____

____

____

Who will I share my success with? ______________________________

What will I do when I reach my goal? How will that make me feel? ______________________________

____

____

____

Date: ________________ Day 81 of 90

I press on toward the goal to win the prize for which God has called. Philippians 3:14

What did I do today—Workout activities?

___

___

___

What did I eat today?

___

___

___

Today's overall grade: ________________

Overall Feedback: ________________

___

___

Father God, I submit my body to You. I pray for strength to honor You through it. Thank You for what you have allowed me to achieve today. Amen.

Journal

What did I do well today? ______________________________

____

____

____

____

What will I do differently tomorrow? ______________________________

____

____

____

____

Who will I share my success with? ______________________________

What will I do when I reach my goal? How will that make me feel? ______________________________

____

____

____

Date: ________________ Day 82 of 90

I press on toward the goal to win the prize for which God has called. Philippians 3:14

What did I do today—Workout activities?

____

____

____

What did I eat today?

____

____

____

Today's overall grade: ________________

Overall Feedback: ______________________________

____

____

Father God, I submit my body to You. I pray for strength to honor You through it. Thank You for what you have allowed me to achieve today. Amen.

Journal

What did I do well today? ______________________________

____

____

____

____

What will I do differently tomorrow? ______________________________

____

____

____

____

Who will I share my success with? ______________________________

What will I do when I reach my goal? How will that make me feel? ______________________________

____

____

____

Date: ________________ Day 83 of 90

I press on toward the goal to win the prize for which God has called. Philippians 3:14

What did I do today—Workout activities?

____

____

____

What did I eat today?

____

____

____

Today's overall grade: ________________

Overall Feedback: ________________________________

____

____

Father God, I submit my body to You. I pray for strength to honor You through it. Thank You for what you have allowed me to achieve today. Amen.

Journal

What did I do well today? ______________________________

____

____

____

____

What will I do differently tomorrow? ______________________________

____

____

____

____

Who will I share my success with? ______________________________

What will I do when I reach my goal? How will that make me feel? ______________________________

____

____

____

Date: ________________ Day 84 of 90

I press on toward the goal to win the prize for which God has called. Philippians 3:14

What did I do today—Workout activities?

____

____

____

What did I eat today?

____

____

____

Today's overall grade: ________________

Overall Feedback: ______________________________

____

____

Father God, I submit my body to You. I pray for strength to honor You through it. Thank You for what you have allowed me to achieve today. Amen.

Journal

What did I do well today? ______________________________

____

____

____

____

What will I do differently tomorrow? ______________________________

____

____

____

____

Who will I share my success with? ______________________________

What will I do when I reach my goal? How will that make me feel? ______________________________

____

____

____

Date: ________________ Day 85 of 90

So God created mankind in His own image. Genesis 1:27

What did I do today—Workout activities?

____

____

____

What did I eat today?

____

____

____

Today's overall grade: ________________

Overall Feedback: ____

____

____

Father God, I submit my body to You. I pray for strength to honor You through it. Thank You for what you have allowed me to achieve today. Amen.

Journal

What did I do well today? ______________________________

____

____

____

____

What will I do differently tomorrow? ______________________________

____

____

____

____

Who will I share my success with? ______________________________

What will I do when I reach my goal? How will that make me feel? ______________________________

____

____

____

Date: ________________ Day 86 of 90

So God created mankind in His own image. Genesis 1:27

What did I do today—Workout activities?

___

___

___

What did I eat today?

___

___

___

Today's overall grade: ________________

Overall Feedback: ________________

___

___

Father God, I submit my body to You. I pray for strength to honor You through it. Thank You for what you have allowed me to achieve today. Amen.

Journal

What did I do well today? ______________________________

____

____

____

____

What will I do differently tomorrow? ______________________________

____

____

____

____

Who will I share my success with? ______________________________

What will I do when I reach my goal? How will that make me feel? ______________________________

____

____

____

Date: ________________ Day 87 of 90

So God created mankind in His own image. Genesis 1:27

What did I do today—Workout activities?

____

____

____

What did I eat today?

____

____

____

Today's overall grade: ________________

Overall Feedback: ____

____

____

Father God, I submit my body to You. I pray for strength to honor You through it. Thank You for what you have allowed me to achieve today. Amen.

Journal

What did I do well today? ______________________________

____

____

____

____

What will I do differently tomorrow? ______________________________

____

____

____

____

Who will I share my success with? ______________________________

What will I do when I reach my goal? How will that make me feel? ______________________________

____

____

____

Date: ________________ Day 88 of 90

So God created mankind in His own image. Genesis 1:27

What did I do today—Workout activities?

____

____

____

What did I eat today?

____

____

____

Today's overall grade: ________________

Overall Feedback: ______________________________

____

____

Father God, I submit my body to You. I pray for strength to honor You through it. Thank You for what you have allowed me to achieve today. Amen.

Journal

What did I do well today? ______________________________

____

____

____

____

What will I do differently tomorrow? ______________________________

____

____

____

____

Who will I share my success with? ______________________________

What will I do when I reach my goal? How will that make me feel? ______________________________

____

____

____

Date: ________________ Day 89 of 90

So God created mankind in His own image. Genesis 1:27

What did I do today—Workout activities?

___

___

___

What did I eat today?

___

___

___

Today's overall grade: ________________

Overall Feedback: ________________

___

___

Father God, I submit my body to You. I pray for strength to honor You through it. Thank You for what you have allowed me to achieve today. Amen.

Journal

What did I do well today? ___

___

___

___

___

What will I do differently tomorrow? ___

___

___

___

___

Who will I share my success with? ___

What will I do when I reach my goal? How will that make me feel? ___

___

___

___

Date: ________________ Day 90 of 90

So God created mankind in His own image. Genesis 1:27

What did I do today—Workout activities?

____

____

____

What did I eat today?

____

____

____

Today's overall grade: ________________

Overall Feedback: ______________________________

____

____

Father God, I submit my body to You. I pray for strength to honor You through it. Thank You for what you have allowed me to achieve today. Amen.

Journal

What did I do well today? ______________________________

____

____

____

____

What will I do differently tomorrow? ______________________________

____

____

____

____

Who will I share my success with? ______________________________

What will I do when I reach my goal? How will that make me feel? ______________________________

____

____

____

90 Day Progress Check

I now have the following

measurements and the following weight:

	Now	+/-
Weight	____________________	____________________
Measurements		
Arms	____________________	____________________
Chest	____________________	____________________
Waist	____________________	____________________
Hips	____________________	____________________
Thighs	____________________	____________________

Journal

What did I do well today? ______________________________

____

____

____

____

What will I do differently tomorrow? ______________________________

____

____

____

____

Who will I share my success with? ______________________________

What will I do when I reach my goal? How will that make me feel? ______________________________

____

____

____

Did I reach my goal? ____

What will I do now that I have reached my goal? What will I do if I did not reach my goal?

____

____

____

____

How do I feel about myself now that I completed these 90 days? ______________________

____

____

____

____

What will I do to maintain what I have achieved? ______________________

____

____

Reflection

Acknowledgements

God, thank You for Your plans for me. Thank You for ***From Fat to Fit in 90 Days, A Fitness Journal,*** and choosing me to complete Your project. I just want to please You, God. Thank You for continuing to anoint me and to invest in me and my gifts, which keep surprising me. Thank You for loving and forgiving me.

Hillary and Nehemiah, thank you for supporting me and my endeavors. Thank you for loving me, especially when I do nothing without a pen and a clipboard, thank you for enduring my late nights, your ideas, the sounding board, the love and the support. Thank you for celebrating our legacy.

To my prayer partners and to my accountability partners, thank you for the long talks and the powerful prayers and the encouragement.

To the readers who this will reach and empower and touch and affect, may these words empower you and help you reach some resolve. May you be inspired to achieve your goals and dreams. May you enhance your relationship with God so that your other relationships will also improve. May you enhance your self-esteem through prayer and study. May you have courage and peace. Share love the best you can until you can share love without reservation.

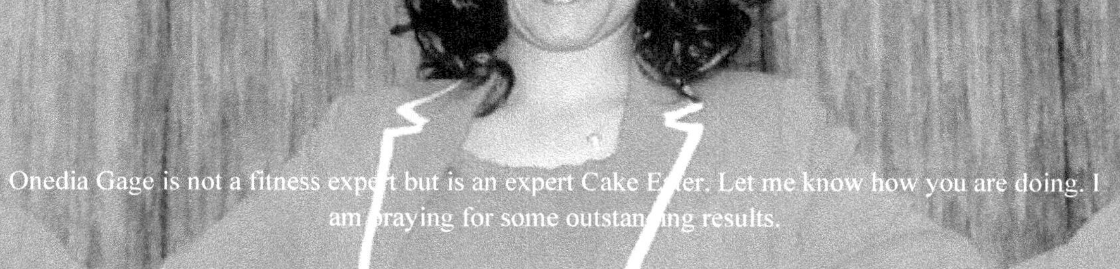

Onedia Gage is not a fitness expert but is an expert Cake Eater. Let me know how you are doing. I am praying for some outstanding results.

Please feel free to contact and share your testimony. onediagage@onediagage.com, or @onediangage (twitter). www.onediagage.com

Blogtalkradio.com/onediagage

Youtube.com/onediagage

Facebook.com/onedia-gage-ministries

MOTIVATIONAL SPEAKER ♦ COACH

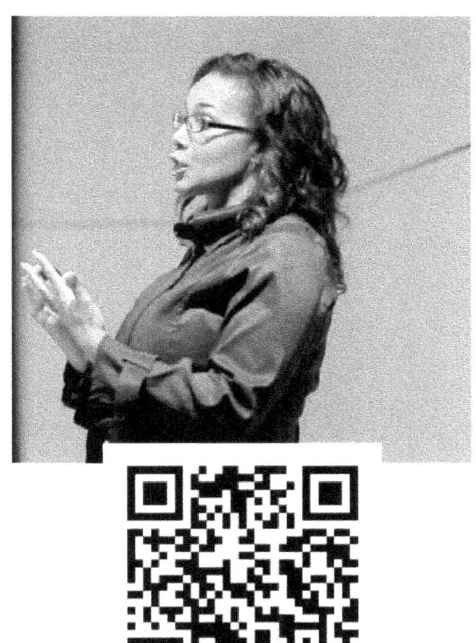

To invite Rev. Gage to preach, teach, and pray, Please contact us at

@onediangage (twitter) ♦ onediagage@onediagage.com ♦ facebook.com/onediagage

youtube.com/onediagage ♦ blogtalkradio.com/onediagage ♦ www.onediagage.com

www.ingramcontent.com/pod-product-compliance
Lightning Source LLC
Chambersburg PA
CBHW080418030426
42335CB00020B/2495
* 9 7 8 1 9 3 9 1 1 9 2 0 9 *